Table Of Contents

Covering My Butt (Legal Junk)

I'll make this fast and easy, if you reuse any of my work in this book you agree to pay me 5,000 times the highest purchase price as a resale based product and agree to cover any legal fees and fees directly or indirectly related to any legal proceedings.

This book is based on my thoughts and my own personal research. They should be used for informational and educational purposes only. As with any decision in life the responsibility is yours to research and seek medical advice before trying anything. You agree to hold me harmless in any result from you attempting to put into action any of the ideas laid out in this book. It is your responsibility to consult with your doctor.

I'll paraphrase this, This book is a collection of my thoughts, findings, and experiences as a personal trainer and someone who studies health related topics. I'll never claim my medical advice will work better than a doctor's, nor can I tell if you are doing an exercise properly. It's up to you to seek out a doctor and trainer and that is not a bad idea!

Pay Attention to the teachings in this book. Occasionally I will recommend a product. Those products are completely optional and are not needed for the principals in this book to work. Again you need to read the Medical disclaimer. Additionally, I may receive compensation if you decide to purchase the product. I have no business relationship with any product or parties recommended in this book, I am solely receiving a commission if you purchase them – I have gone through them myself however, and have no issue putting my name behind them!

I'll say it again in terms my, well I'll dumb it down to be nice ***DOING ANYTHING THAT WILL AFFECT YOUR HEALTH WITHOUT TALKING TO A LICENSED DOCTOR FIRST IS FLAT OUT STUPID! ASSUME YOU COULD DIE (or get better, not a good 50/50 chance game if you ask me). THIS INCLUDES POPPING AN AMINO ACID SUPPLEMENT!***

Now that my butt is covered let's get into this!

Introduction, Sort Of...

In life, we sometimes make mistakes by not fully understanding something and instead going by our assumptions. I am just as guilty of this as you probably are, and I have been wrong as well as missed out on some great opportunities. I have also been let down due to assumptions more than I'd like to admit. This book is catered to, what I have realized through conversations, the misconception of amino acids!

Many have thought amino acids to be something that only those involved with bodybuilding or extreme fitness athletes worry about. You may or may not realize it, however amino acids play an intricate part of your life and daily functions as well!

So what are amino acids seeing I now have your attention? Amino acids, and here's where you can slap your forehead and say "opps", are a chemical unit sort of building block that help make up proteins. That's not all, amino acids are also the end product that comes from hydrolysis (protein digestion).

As in another book I wrote, **Phytonutrient Superfoods**, amino acids have some similarities with other nutritional substances, sugars as well as fatty acids. They also contain a huge difference and have something that sugars and fatty acids do not which helps with their abilities as well as chemical processes. The chemical or element they have that fatty acids and sugars don't is nitrogen. In fact, amino acids are believed to be roughly 16 percent nitrogen containing.

Are you still stuck on the fact that protein is something only needed by athletes as well as body builders? I already told you you should we need them, but I also reminded you we shouldn't fall victim to misconceptions or assumptions, good point. So we should stop the topic there, right? Of course not, besides I talk way too much and you invested in this book! So let's get into why proteins are important.

Amino Acids Make Up Protein, But Why Is Protein so Important?

Although we now know amino acids are the building blocks of protein, what do we know about protein (aside from the fact that not only bodybuilders need it)? The question of why proteins are so important is a great one, let's start exploring the answer!

Actually, proteins are extremely important! Protein creates and provides a structure for every single living thing on Earth (just in case you believe in aliens, the Martian kind, I figured I'd include you too because I'm sometimes politically correct). Everything that is alive regardless of size needs protein equally. It doesn't matter if the species is a massive blue whale or an itty bitty amoeba, they both have the same need for protein. Every living thing is composed of protein and it's the protein through chemical reactions (there's a whole lot of different forms of proteins) that sustain life!

Protein sustains life? Yeah, I swear it does! It's a known fact we need oxygen to survive, and we need food to nourish ourselves. Not to be gross, but do you breathe out oxygen? Do you poop out the same food you just ate (if you do there is a mega problem going on inside of you)? Wasn't trying to be gross, and if you got grossed out thank God I didn't add pictures there. What I was getting at is that we consume things and they become altered in our body through chemical processes and different functions. Proteins are behind all of that!.

Because my mother always said I should have been a corporate lawyer, how about I give you another argument to why we need protein in case having it sustain life wasn't a solid reason? Sorry about the long sentences, however I digress and will ask what makes up the majority of our body, first and second place. If you're stuck after saying water, I'll tell you. Aside from water (having the majority and winning first place) our bodies are primarily made up of protein! How so? Our muscles, tendons, vital organs (and even the non-vital ones), ligaments, hair, nails, and glands are all made up of protein.

Protein also makes up many vital fluids in our body (have you ever heard about proteins being checked in different medical tests, say in blood or urine for example). What about bones, they need calcium more than anything right? WRONG! Protein is also instrumental in the growth of healthy bones!

Let's keep going a bit more on the processes that protein is the backbone of. Have you ever heard of hormones and enzymes? Guess what, those two things that catalyze and control our bodily processes and functions are proteins.

Protein also helps to keep in check your pH balance (and unlike the deodorant commercial suggests, men and women need proper pH balance). If you're not sure the importance of this, I highly suggest you learn the importance from 2 great and short books Naturally Improve Diabetes and How To Reverse Diabetes.

Want one more tell tale sign that proteins are important and help sustain life? Do you remember when I gave the poop example above? It's proteins that help the nutrients process and make up the change between lymph's, various tissues, as well as blood that the nutrients go through. In a weird sense you could think of proteins as being the machines at an automated processing plant.

Before I go on and really start to introduce the shining star of this short book, let's digress to a statement I made earlier and actually build on it. Remember where I said protein sustains life about a page or two ago? Life is created by God (in my faith, no sarcasm I am faithful and a Believer), but according to science it's DNA. Do you know that DNA is actually an internal blueprint on how to make that cell's protein? If you didn't know, no you know (I grew up watching the real G.I. Joe cartoon. Let's jump into amino acids, shall we?

<u>Introducing Amino Acids!</u>

So, we've discovered that protein is some extremely important stuff, right? If you need to, I'll wait, go to the beginning of the book and reread what makes up proteins (if you're lazy or wise, just look at the title of the chapter again). So which one is more important nutritionally? Amino acids make up protein, amino acids, rather than protein, are the essential nutrient out of the two.

So what do amino acids do? Amino acids act is an extremely great variety of roles, and just like phytonutrients (which I cover in **Phytonutrient Superfoods**) are similar yet completely different. Let's get a better understanding of the previous statement shall we?

Some amino acids combine to form the bodies proteins, hence the label of protein's building blocks. But that's not all amino acids, and that's certainly not to say the other aminos aren't equally important. Some amino acids for example some act to support your metabolic functions.

A really cool job of aminos (I got tired of seeing amino acids typed everywhere, aminos are the same thing, just me adding some variety) deals with something powerful to you and its reliance on aminos! The heart, yes in a sense, but I am talking about the brain! Here's how, some of the amino acids act precursors of neurotransmitters. This means they help with the information that is getting passed from cell to cell in your body. Without these amino acids, your brain cannot send or receive complete information.

Your body must consider amino acids important as they have a VIP pass when it comes to getting through your blood - brain barrier. What this barrier does is it blocks almost everything from entering your brain as a defense against toxins, think of the aminos that do this as your brains special messenger (or at least the driving force behind it).

How about checking into the functions of amino acids in another cool and extremely different way? Well, you're still going to be reading this but I was talking about seeing what else they can do. We talked about metabolism and how amino acids help with metabolic functions, right?

Amino acids are also good friends or helpers to vitamins and minerals. The aminos (some) help them do their jobs even better, for example they could help pro-vitamin A convert more efficiently into vitamin A.

The paragraph above sounds like vitamins and minerals are useless unless we have amino acids, right? Let's look at Taurine. Sure we can absorb and have these important things, minerals and vitamins, assimilate into our body. But without adequate levels of taurine, we could still become iron deficient (no fun!).

Do you know how some of the elderly start to develop depressive states more often, and are also more prone to other neurological problems? There are a few studies that may have found a common denominator that could correlate something missing in them with those mental issues. Know what it is? If you said taurine, you're wrong. There's a good chance they are however missing an amino from the group of tyrosine, tryptophan, phenylalanine, or histidine.

They could also be missing branch-chained amino acids in their body. Branched-chain amino acids, what are they? Don't worry about that yet, we'll get to them when I start going over ALL of the amino acids!

Did you know some amino acids are even used in hospitals? That must mean they're pretty important I'd say! In fact, sometimes in hospitals branched-chain aminos are used to help treat things such as infection or other severe traumas!

How Many Amino Acids Are There?

There's hundreds, maybe even thousands of different proteins in the body, right? Did you know they come from a whopping 25 different amino acids? Yep, there are 25 different amino acids, but did you know that about 80% of them come from our very own liver? Dead serious, no kidding! Those are called the non-essential amino acids.

20 percent of the amino acids we need to survive do however have to come from our diet. So whereas we don't necessarily need protein from our diet, we do need to consume 20% of the amino acids from diet.

Do you know what these amino acids are called? They're essential amino acids, right! To be a nice guy, I'll give you a list of BOTH the essential and nonessential amino acids! I'm also going to give you some information on what amino acids do and how we can get them into our diet!

The essential amino acids that we have to get through dietary means are:

- Histidine
- Isoleucine
- Leucine
- Lysine
- Methionine
- Phenylalanine
- Threonine
- Tryptophan
- Valine

The nonessential amino acids that our body can produce without needing supplementation (for the most part) are:

- Alanine
- Arginine
- Asparagine
- Aspartic Acid
- Citrulline
- Cysteine
- Cystine
- Gamma-Aminobutyric Acid (GABA)
- Glutamic Acid
- Glutamine
- Glycine
- Ornithine
- Proline
- Serine
- Taurine
- Tyrosine

Want to know something confusing about the nonessential amino acids (yes, besides their name you silly sarcastic reader you)? Just because they're nonessential doesn't take away from their importance and it doesn't mean their nonessential. They perform certain roles that are imperative to everyday life, function, and even composition (how we're made, not like a Mozart piece).

Something else that's confusing about the nonessential amino acids is their classification. They are nonessential initially, however they can actually turn into an essential amino acid!

I should have put this one in first as it is definitely far more confusing than the above tidbit of information. An example of this would be if you don't take in enough methionine or phenylalanine, cysteine and tyrosine would now become additional essential amino acids. Why is this you may be asking? Well simple, it is because methionine and phenylalanine actually make the non essential aminos cysteine and tyrosine!

Let's talk really fast about the dependence on different proteins on amino acids. Assembling the aminos we've discussed to help create various proteins (again, building blocks) is not a one shot deal and in fact happens very regularly. If your reserves of enzyme proteins are running low for example, your body is going to start creating more. If you need more cells made because your other cells are banged up or depleted, your body uses amino acids to help the proteins form more cells. Keep this constant automation or clockwork in mind for the next paragraph as I discuss the importance of amino acids in your body.

This is going to show you on a micro level how important amino acids are in that a shortage of even one single (not simple as they are complex items) amino acid, the clock work stops working. The automation becomes screwed up and the potential for DNA type damage can become real.

If an amino acid isn't there or is severely hindered to a state that it is insufficient, the protein type dependant on it will not form! What happens now is your nitrogen balance is going to be completely off where you body is accumulating more nitrogen than it can assimilate - not good.

Another essential aspect to the essential amino acids is that they all have to "meet" or be in your body at the same time. If they're not, the other amino acids aren't going to be properly utilized, they can't (if you're asking why - they just can't. There's a lot of scientific words and I've been looking into that because it's fascinating for years, we're talking extremely complex stuff) work. What happens in a state like this is an emergency, because now the nitrogen balance in your body is going to be completely screwed up again. What else happens? Stunted growth, indigestion, depression, and other nasty things happen because the vital proteins are now being created at a drastically slow pace.

How can a miracle like the human body let something like this happen? Very easy, there are a wide variety of factors that play into this, even if you are eating a God inspired diet (maybe not, because then you'd have Divine Intervention and you'd probably work perfectly). A well-balanced diet containing all of the essential amino acids may not even be able to stop this due to the factors I'm about to mention.

If your ability to absorb food is messed up, you can see the issue discussed above take place. The same thing goes if you have lower levels of vitamin C in your diet as this can affect how your lower intestine absorbs or takes in the amino acids. If you're not getting enough vitamin b6 your amino acids will not get transported properly. Think of b6 sort of like a limo for a rich and famous person, without their chauffeur they are screwed as they can't drive that well. Vitamin b6 is needed for the transportation of amino acids through your body.

Although I mentioned you could have a great diet with the above issues still taking place, you still need a well balanced diet.

If your diet fails to provide an adequate amount of amino acids (don't worry, they're tasteless - it's the food they're in you have to worry about) sooner or later you'll end up with some form of a physical issue or disorder. Does that mean you run out and eat a ton of protein (this is especially true for the vegans as well as vegetarians)? No way, in fact I'd even go as far say saying don't (even though I'm not licensed in any field of medicine or nutrition, I've studied this stuff for years out of interest and know it inside and out, but [yeah it's a disclaimer] you're always going to want to run things like this to your doctor or nutritionist) even think about it.

There is a great reason you don't want to isn't because you'll end up looking like a bodybuilder which we mentioned and is commonly thought to have a high protein diet.

You don't want to run out and start scarfing tons of protein because it really isn't all that healthy of an idea. Why not, after all that's mainly how we get amino acids right?

Here's why you don't want to go nuts with your protein intake, it puts a ton of stress on your kidneys as well as your liver. Yeah, the liver that is nice and makes the nonessential amino acids for it. Let's put this into perspective with an example shall we?

Think back to a time when you completely snapped and lost it on someone. You didn't go irate out of the blue, right (if you did you may have a serious, or at the minimum [no baby mom jokes although I could throw one here], mental or personality disorder)? There were things that led up to it, maybe a lot of pressure to perform at work, exhaustion, upsetting items, or just too much of life at once right? A build up of stressors caused you to become the Jerk of the Year even if only for a few moments.

The example above is the same thing that can happen to your liver and kidneys. Protein is a great, awesome, and essential component for your survival.

But remember the saying your mom told you growing up, "too much of anything is never a good thing". The saying from mom holds true even with protein. Want to know what happens and why too much protein is bad? I'll explain (especially since my post workout protein consumption plummeted after learning this).

Your liver and kidneys take in and put out. A large amount, some say it nears or exceeds (we're not robots so I take this with a grain of salt - no nutritional pun intended) half, of dietary protein is turned into glucose. How? The liver does it. This isn't so bad actually, because that glucose is used to give your cells energy kicks! When your cells are done with their energy kick, they create ammonia. The cleaning ammonia? No, it's bodily ammonia. And it's not good - at all.

Actually the excess ammonia is very toxic for your body. What happens next is your body starts fighting back (sort of like the fight or flight idea discussed in Mind Games : Mental Survival And Stress' Effects On The Body) by bringing your liver into the issue full fledged and turning that ammonia into urea.

So we're safe now, right? NOPE! This is where your body calls your kidneys in. The urea travels by bloodstream to your kidney headquarters (sorry for the geekiness, it seems like we're going to war though, in a sense, doesn't it) where they filter and excrete it. High urea levels can cause inflamed kidneys; you don't want to keep beating your kidneys for a long time trust me!

The Amino Acids: Introducing Each One!

We've been talking about protein, consumption, and the importance of amino acids for a while now, why don't we start introducing each individual amino acid now? Sound fun? Let's get to know them!

You'll more than likely notice some amino acids have more information than others, and that's okay. The reason for this is that I, as well as science, know a lot more about some amino acids than others. Does this mean the ones with less information are less important? Of course not, we already discussed what happens when one amino acid is off. Some just have better stories for a lack of words, but they're all equally as important to another.

I forgot to mention, I'll be covering the amino acids from nonessential (A-T) and then the essential aminos (A-V). Is that a typo? No, if you remember form 2 pages ago tyrosine is the last nonessential amino acid alphabetically while valine is the last essential amino alphabetically.

<u>Meet Alanine</u>

Your first impression of this word may have you thinking it is the name Alan in some European dialect of some sort. Actually, this amino acid plays some important roles so we can't really goof on its name too much (we can but of course that's not very friendly).

Alanine plays a pivotal role in helping your body transport nitrogen from the peripheral tissues (tissue that goes around something, I.E. nervous system, skeletal, etc.) to your liver. That's not all it helps to do or create, alanine also aids in helping with metabolizing the carb/sugar glucose (a simple carb that once broken down the body uses for energy).

Well and dandy, right? There's something else you need to know about alanine, it acts as a protector or buffer as well! When your muscle protein is broken down to supply energy on a cellular level, it releases toxic substances. This is when your body needs some quick energy bursts such as with aerobic exercise.

Remember before when we were talking about the adverse effect of amino acid levels, or when aminos were not hanging out in sufficient levels in your body? If you're lacking on your naturally (which form of amino is naturally made? Great memory, the nonessentials!) made tyrosine and phenylalanine and have higher than normal alanine levels you may feel tired. This amino acid (problem) combination can results in something along the lines of chronic fatigue as well as potentially the Epstein-Barr viral infection. Not fun stuff let me tell you.

I almost forgot something, have you ever heard of coenzyme A? What about pantothenic acid? They're both extremely important in your body, actually they are both vital catalysts for your body and health as well as wellbeing. What am I getting at? A form of alanine (beta-alanine) is a massive component of their makeup and structure! Pretty neat huh? Who would have thought making fun of this European sounding amino acid meant you were dissing something you need for survive?

One last thing I want to talk about, and it'll be quick, is a study that was published (there were a few, this particular study I found really interesting) regarding diabetics. Do you know how many diabetics will eat a snack before bed to prevent hypoglycemia during the night? It turns out that taking a simple oral dose of L-alanine may be more effective than that nighttime snack! The results showed a lot of promise however were inconclusive. If you're diabetic, why don't you ask your endocrinologist what they've heard about this? If you're trying to lose weight this could be a better option for you!

Arginine, Popular In Sports Crucial For Health!

Another odd sounding amino acid here, this one is named arginine and if you were impressed with what alanine can do, this one will knock your socks off!

Do you know what a retardant is? Think of a flame retardant for example, they are sprayed on things to slow the spread of fire on clothing right? In the woods ditches or gullies are dug to help create a man made (as if chemicals aren't) fire retardant. Think of mental retardation (don't make fun of them, no jokes for this one), what is it? It's a slow development, especially on the cognitive and mental aspects, right? Arginine does the same thing!

How does arginine act as a retardant you may be wondering and why is slowing things down cooler than diabetics needing a snack before bed? What if I told you it slowed down the growth rate of cancer and tumor cells? Dead serious, oh you're interested now? It does this by enhancing your natural immune function; it does this by making your thymus gland a little larger and far more active. It may sound scary, but guess what your thymus gland does; it releases T cells (T lymphocytes) which are extremely important in the function and maintenance of a healthy immune system.

Who else could benefit from have a more active thymus gland, what about people with autoimmune issues, sort of like AIDS? Will arginine cure AIDS? No, but if it helps prolong life by again retarding the spread or severity of

AIDS by increasing the overall immune punches your T Cells have, you'd be in better shape.

That's not all that arginine does for your body, that's not even the start. Maybe you're not worried about cancer or AIDS (nothing wrong with being celibate, maybe I have a nun reading this), so you could be wondering if arginine does anything for you. No problem does your liver work and if so would you want it to keep working? Arginine helps in this area as well.

I consider arginine to be a "child" amino acid in the regard to liver. A good child helps their parents, right? Arginine helps the liver, which makes it (see my "child" amino relation? Parents make child, child helps parent and liver makes arginine, arginine helps liver?) sort of like the liver's child in a freakish way. Arginine helps the liver in a few ways. It helps with liver disorders like a fatty liver (making it easier to filter and produce) as well as with cirrhosis. How does it do this stuff? Do you remember when I mentioned ammonia and how it turns into urea? What arginine does is it aids in the detoxification of the liver by going after and neutralizing the ammonia.

Arginine is really all encompassing if you ask me, not only does it help a vital organ and promote a super powered immune system, arginine is also great helper when it comes to muscle metabolism! Think of arginine as sort of a trash truck for your muscles, here's how it does that. Imagine a big pile of trash that needs to go somewhere. You'd start loading the trash truck so it doesn't create a massive pile and in turn result in problems, like a bad smell right? Arginine takes nitrogen and helps store it and when not needed, it dumps the nitrogen through excretion.

Helping maintain that nitrogen balance in your body, arginine does more than just getting rid of the waste; sometimes in a balanced equation you need more of something to keep the balance, right? It could also help you after surgery as it can improve the function of cells in your lymphatic system.

Are you wondering if we're done with arginine yet, I mean I can't blame you we've already touched on some real important factors. No, we're actually really just getting started with the topic (or conversation if you'd rather use that word. Here's something for all the vain people out there, or athletes working to alter their physique. Arginine also can help with weight loss!

Arginine can help with weight loss, if your mouth is on the floor and eyes wide open keep reading (and if you didn't brush your teeth take 5 and knock that out, or close your mouth). Let me backtrack a bit (especially since I was a personal trainer), you're not losing weight but you could lose fat. We already mentioned how arginine helps move nitrogen around when you have the stuff pumping through your muscles after they break right? Arginine also helps to rebuild that muscle mass slightly and can reduce area body fat.

What else is arginine important in, how about maintaining order in a household that would see some dangerous deficiencies if it was missing? There are functions that we need to maintain great health, and if arginine is not sufficiently being produced (what does it become? An ESSENTIAL amino acid, right) you will start seeing the negative effects. Lipid metabolism in the liver (fat), insulin production, glucose tolerance (start thinking blood sugar issues) are some of the functions that could go into a nosedive if arginine is lacking in your body.

Speaking of arginine lacking, do you know there are some who genetically have a problem producing arginine? Infants and toddlers can naturally have much lower levels as arginine production doesn't come fully into the picture at birth and slowly begins to increase later through growth. Babies will have some arginine; it's just that the levels they produce are more than likely going to be inadequate to keep up with the demands of the body. This is why you'll notice some foods, such as soybean, dairy, carob, and other food sources recommended during breastfeeding.

I say during breastfeeding because it is not encouraged for mother's to supplement with l-arginine while they are breastfeeding.

Babies aren't the only ones who shouldn't have l-arginine supplements, people with oral herpes may want to look into lysine as compared to arginine, especially in the diet. It's not just oral herpes either but a wide variety of viral infections as arginine could promote growth in the viral cells making them tougher to treat.

Now we're done with arginine, and we're going to start touching on one of the shortest bits of information about any amino acids.

Asparagine, Our First Dino Sounding Amino

Asparagine has some of the fewest benefits of the amino acids, but you need to realize small things come in small packages (like my fiance at the time of this writing, even though she won't grow anymore we'll be married if you're reading this after 2015)? This is especially true of asparagine.

This particular amino acid is a true amino acid as it is created from the next one we're going to cover. What's an important job of asparagine? How about being needed to maintain balance in the central nervous system? It's sort of like being the appointment setter for a really popular and needed government official (bad example, they hardly show up to work, ha-ha). If this amino isn't fully sufficient you could be way too calm or extremely nervous, and both aren't all that desirable.

That's not all that asparagine does though, when it returns to aspartic acid it releases energy. What sort of energy does it release you may be asking? Energy that the brain and metabolism both use for metabolism!

Lastly, this amino promotes the process where one amino acid turns into or converts into another amino inside the liver. I'd say this amino is pretty important, wouldn't you?

Aspartic Acid

Aspartic Acid aside from being the amino acid that helps create (before it turns back into aspartic acid) asparagine it also focuses on increasing stamina. Because of this, having solid levels of this amino acid could mean that the chances of you getting depression or chronic fatigue are much lower. In fact, chronic fatigue could actually result from your body having low levels of aspartic acid!

Like it's quasi-offspring asparagine, aspartic acid is also beneficial and needed by the brain as it can aid in reducing the occurrence or severity of neural and brain disorders. In fact, there's a correlation here with neural and brain disorders specifically epilepsy as well as certain depressive disorders.

In a decent amount of epilepsy findings when looking at the blood/brain makeup it is found that some of these individuals have abnormally high levels of aspartic acid. On the other hand, a good amount of people falling into certain depression types have very low levels of this particular amino.

Let's talk about the similarities of a few amino acids, specifically arginine as well as aspartic acid, they both share a common benefit. Aspartic acid just like arginine helps the liver by getting rid of some ammonia that's not needed, as well as very toxic.

Aspartic acid acts as a team player as well when it comes to toxins and their removal from the bloodstream. Aspartic acid joins forces with a few other amino acids and plays a pivotal role in helping form the molecules that absorb the toxins I just mentioned.

There's some other nifty benefits to having a partnership inside your body with this helpful amino. If you put metal in water, you'll notice that it doesn't suspend well and sort of sinks to the bottom right?

Minerals are sort of like metals as they come from ores, and in turn like to hang out in your intestinal lining, which is better than being in your bloodstream, right? Not so much, in fact some minerals in proper levels are great for your health! This is where aspartic acid comes in and helps to move these beneficial and heavy minerals into your bloodstream and other cells.

Aspartic acid also does other things on a cellular level, it helps them function. Something else aspartic acid helps out is the functioning of RNA and DNA (your body's blueprints) which carry all your genetic markers and other crucial information.

Proteins, specific proteins to be exact, also get a helping hand from aspartic acid. Aspartic acid helps with the production of immunoglobulins and antibodies (these are immune system proteins).

Sounds like this amino play a pivotal role, doesn't it?

Citrulline The Promoter

Dieting? If so, you may want to cross your fingers and hope
your body is pumping decent levels of citrulline through
your body, know why? Citrulline (which I should say is
created from ornithine), although it isn't a fat eater like
other amino acids plays a huge role in promoting energy.

Aside from being an amino that helps with your energy
levels, citrulline also stimulates your immune system.
When citrulline is metabolized by your body, we get
another amino acid, l-arginine.

Short and sweet. I almost forgot to throw this in here, being
a liver based amino (citrulline is normally found hanging
out in there), also helps to detoxify that nasty stuff called
ammonia.

Meet the Siamese Amino Twins!

Cysteine and Cystine are considered, to me at least, I've never seen it described this way elsewhere, to be Siamese amino acids. I take that label from Siamese twins, which as you know are twins that are physically joined together. Every single cystine molecule contains two cysteine molecules, pretty interesting ey?

The reason (not the scientific reason, but it goes with the easy reading of this book) that these separate (in a technical term, we already know they're joined) aminos are joined is because cysteine never makes it mind up!

It's a very unstable amino acid and can convert into l-cystine very easily, actually both of them can convert into the other just as easily, but that's just a little factoid, let's look at what they can do.

Cysteine helps with the production of collagen and promotes the texture and how elastic your skin is. The elderly typically don't have strong or high levels of collagen or this amino acid and thus have the wrinkly and flabby skin.

Do you remember how I mentioned that proteins and enzymes are made up of amino acids? The proteins in your hair, nails, as well as skin contain a protein called alpha-keratin. It's not the only protein in there, but it's the most active for a lack of words, and it contains a ton of the amino acid cysteine!

Cysteine isn't just a confused amino acid that plays with beauty based proteins. Actually if you're not careful and overly powerful cysteine will knock you out (that is if you are radiation damage or a free radical). In fact, cysteine is one of the best free radical destroyers your body has! If you're supplementing with this amino acid make sure you take it with vitamin E and selenium as it works best when taken in combination with those.Along the same lines as killing free radicals and protecting against radiation damage, cysteine helps you detoxify toxins.

Do you remember how citrulline helps the body by promoting energy production? This amino can help you in your dieting ways too as it helps with the promotion of fat burning as well as muscle growth and building!

Although this amino is "confused" we know far more about its benefits and workings than we do with its Siamese amino twin cystine. We do know something about it; the N-acetyl form is extremely effective against the effects of radiation and chemotherapy.

Want to know something else really cool about N-acetylcysteine? It can help promote and increase glutathione levels in bone marrow, the kidneys, your liver, as well as your lungs and has anti aging effects attributed to it!

If supplementing with cysteine, you're going to want to make sure you're also taking in 2 B vitamins (B6 & B12) as well as folate to ensure the cysteine is being synthesized. If you have a chronic illness of some kind, you may need to take upwards of 1,000 mg's 3 times daily for a month straight! Just make sure you remember to run this past your doctor as they know best when it comes to sickness and supplements!

<u>GABA!!!!!!!!!</u>

Aside from having a cool sounding name (say it with me, GABA) gamma-aminobutyric acid is pretty helpful in your body as well. Like a few of the other amino acids, this particular one acts as a neurotransmitter inside of your central nervous system.

Actually, without GABA your brain isn't able to function properly (maybe it's GABA in the morning rather than coffee you need? No, I agree it's definitely java) and is not able to metabolize!

The way GABA works is slightly different than the other neurotransmitters, this amino actually acts as a "cell whisperer" and makes sure your cells are not over firing and in turn screwing up the messages.

It basically decreases the neuron activity which is why some believe this amino acid may be beneficial to individuals with ADD and ADHD although most of the studies I've seen on that idea have promise, none have any conclusive information.

Now we're going to start hitting some cooler information about GABA, guess what drug it acts like? Valium and Librium where it can literally calm your body down! It acts in a way where it acts as a cover for your neuroreceptors so they aren't getting your bodies stress messages! To go along with this, GABA has also been used in some cases to treat epilepsy as well as hypertension (I can attest to the latter!).

Into sex and growth hormones? You may, in case of that, be interested to know that GABA can help with a decreased sex drive, especially if due to stress, and promote human growth hormone (tell the PED popping baseball players that one!)!

Again, like other amino acids, too much of a good thing can be bad and in this case even cause seizures. Do I need to tell you to run supplementing with this past your doctor again or do you remember you need to first?

Glutamic Acid - Comes Before GABA - Really!

Glutamic Acid acts sort of like a parent to GABA, do you see the similarities in them (as far as their name?). This amino actually does the opposite of GABA in that it acts as an excitatory neurotransmitter. Can you guess what that means? Either way you paid for this book so I'll make sure you know, that means (and remember it acts as the opposite of GABA does) it excites your neurons in the central nervous system, making them actually over fire! This amino doesn't stay in its form though, it actually converts into GABA or glutamine (coming up next).

Remember how we had an amino acid act as having a VIP pass to get past your blood-brain barrier? This amino acid has a VIP pass as well as it helps to transport potassium past that barrier as well as into your spinal column. Your brain can also use smaller amounts of glutamic acid as a source of fuel as well.

Metabolism is important when it comes to needs of amino acids, and with glutamic acid that's no different. Glutamic acid helps your body metabolizes fats and sugars into energy.

Again, like other amino acids, glutamic acid helps to detoxify ammonia from your body by picking up itty bitty left over nitrogen atoms, which spawns yet another amino acid! Did you guess glutamine (good job paying attention)? You're right! We'll cover glutamine in a few moments, I want to tell you a few other important tidbits about glutamic acid.

Did you know that mental retardation can be helped? Glutamic acid does that slightly, in fact it is also beneficial for people with personality disorders and helping with childhood behavioral issues (no, it will not make your children listen the first time).

Be Careful though, especially if you are like me and allergic to MSG. One of the salts inside of glutamic acid contains monosodium glutamate. Let's take a peek at glutamine shall we?!

Glutamine Says "I'm the Most Popular"

This amino acid is probably, actually in a healthy individual it is, the most prevalent and abundant amino in your muscles. This amino is also a bonafide brain food as it has no issue passing the blood-brain barrier and the brain gobbles it up as a fuel source.

The brain (when glutamine is eaten by it) turns this amino back into glutamic acid (because glutamine passes into the brain due to free numbers and the brain likes it more [not really, I made that last part about liking it better up]) and puts it right to work helping the cerebral. Glutamine also increases GABA.

Glutamine does a ton more important (if you like life) tasks as well. This amino is the main (or basis) of the building blocks for RNA and DNA synthesis.

We've gone over nitrogen quite a few times, and now we're going to go over it some more, and you're about to see a real important feature of glutamine. Glutamine is like other aminos in that it contains nitrogen, but this is where it differs. Glutamine actually contains two nitrogen atoms!

When glutamine is created, it helps to remove toxic ammonia from the tissues, and none is more important than brain tissue! Back to nitrogen, it also helps your nitrogen transport from one location to another.

With glutamine we know that it is abundant and the most prevalent amino acid in the muscles and body right? Where this comes in extremely helpful is in the need for skeletal muscle. It is also imperative at muscle wasting prevention that is normally seen with diseases such as cancer and AIDs, and even situations such as prolonged bed rest.

Have you ever heard of a state of "fight or flight"? That's when absolute stress is taking over your body, and your muscles in turn release up to one third of it's glutamine stores. In other situations of prolonged stress or illness can lead to the loss of skeletal muscle, guess what…. if you have enough glutamine in your muscles this loss can be thwarted!

Do you know how there are warnings of liver damage of prolonged, and even non regular, use of acetaminophen? Glutamine helps protect your liver against this as well so you don't overdose.

If you're dieting or trying to rid your sweet tooth or quit the booze, you're going to want to talk to your doctor about supplementing with l-glutamine as well. Oh, you want to know right, I got it. It's because glutamine can decrease sugar cravings as well as decreasing your desire for alcohol.

<u>Glycine, Another Retardant!</u>

Glycine acts as another retardant however it goes right after the muscles, in a good way. It helps to retard muscle degeneration by adding more of a substance (which isn't an amino, but is found in us naturally) called creatine. Creatine is important in the construction of DNA as well as RNA, but it's not more important than the amino acids (especially since it relies on them to be added in higher levels to reduce or retard muscular degeneration [wasting]}.

Something I personally find interesting about this amino acid is that it does something cool by improving glucose storage. What this does is that it frees up glucose for energy use.

Here's something important, other amino acids (nonessential) rely on this amino for proper synthesis. It's not just aminos that rely on glycine for synthesis it is also a variety of bile acids as well as nucleic acids.

Glycine is also used in a lot of top shelf (or popular for a nonalcoholic reference) gastric antacids. Why is this? It's because of the fact inside of the fact you're going to find very high concentrations inside of the skin as well as other connective tissues. What this does is it helps to promote repair of damaged tissues as well as promoting healing, which from what i understand is always very appreciated.

Glycine is also something needed for a properly functioning central nervous system and even another cool thing, a healthy prostate!

Like many other amino acids help to fight chronic fatigue issues, this amino in much higher levels can actually cause it.

Ornithine (Fat Fears It And Growth Hormone Loves It)

Our world is becoming more obese, and it appears everywhere you look people have extra fat that they're holding onto for no good reason. Are you one of the many of Americans, or anywhere in the world for that matter, that wishes you could seemingly get rid of this extra fat instead of storing it? What about growth hormone?

Growth hormone, if you are an athlete especially, isn't the best way to go as far as supplements are concerned. In fact, it's illegal to use in many sports (especially baseball), but it helps greatly to get rid of extra body fat! What are we to do?! How about we make it ourselves, in fact the amino acid I'm covering right here and right now briefly is fully capable of helping to release growth hormone! This is the real human growth hormone.

If you combine things in life, you could get a far better effect, right? The growth hormone is helped to be released by ornithine, and if you combine ornithine with carnitine as well as arginine you get, well a fat burning beast!

If you want a properly working immune system, much of my studies into this topic have been conclusive you need some ornithine (along with other key amino acids that we've covered). The same goes for your liver function.

Aside from helping the liver detoxify ammonia, ornithine has also been known to aid it in liver regeneration. Liver regeneration is a fancy way of saying renew or "bring back" liver functions that may have been hampered due to chronic disease or illness.

Something else you should know about this dinosaur sounding amino acid is that it is extremely beneficial in helping tissue heal and repaired itself. If you don't know why, that's because ornithine is found in high concentrations in skin as well as your connective tissues. That makes sense, right?

<u>Proline, Nature's Botox?</u>

Remember when we touched on collagen briefly, and we discussed how it was important in keeping you looking young and vibrant. We also mentioned that it helped keep your skin tight and would help you not look elderly (not the botox elderly, I'm talking about the skinny but droopy the dog looking elderly). A lot of that has to do with collagen production, and this is where our next amino acid comes into the conversation. We're going to shoot over some benefits of proline!

The way proline helps you not look as aged or on your way to droopy cheek syndrome is by improving your skin texture through the aforementioned collagen production. That's not the only improvement based quality of proline, not by far!

Proline can also aid your body in another aging factor, your joints (as well as tendons and heart muscles among other things). It does this by working in harmony with vitamin C (thought it was just good for the sniffles did you? No no!) and together are able to strengthen your joints, tendons, and heart tissue!

Proline is also able to help your body produce fit, or healthy, connective tissues (which we just mentioned, I wanted to put it in another way for you to take in).

<u>Your Body's Handyman – Serine</u>

Serine sound very similar to something that could be a recreational drug, doesn't it? Drugs are normally bad for your body, but serine on the other hand has some extremely important roles.

One of the roles that I found interesting with serine is your muscle health. It's known that the nonessential amino acid serine helps promote muscle growth which makes me wonder, and you should too, seeing I haven't read much into my question if you could turn around and say in theory serine helps promote the abundance of glutamine in our bodies? You'll wonder that because you certainly remember glutamine is the most abundant amino acids in our muscle tissue, right?

The last amino acid we mentioned, ornithine, was instrumental at helping your body release growth hormone to "shed" extra fat, remember? This amino called serine does something, well it's not similar - at all, similar where it is brought into the "fat" conversation. Serine is known to help your body metabolize fats, but more important fatty acids (the good fats) and turn them into energy.

If you've noticed so far, many of these amino acids hold more than 1 job, and serine is no different. Serine is also a protector, but not so much for your liver. Serine helps to "sheath" your nerve fibers. While we're on nerve why don't I also throw it in there that some brain proteins are comprised of serine?

I just mentioned nerves, serine helps another component of our bodies, cell membranes as well as DNA and RNA. It helps your DNA and RNA (cell building blocks) to function properly and aids in the formation of your cell's membranes! Cool right?

If you want to make sure you have a great diet consisting of B vitamins, but need a good reason serine production will give you that reason! In fact, even though your body can make serine from glycine, you're going to need adequate levels of two specific B vitamins, b3 and b6, as well as folic acid for the internal creation of serine to take place.

Serine is not just a muscle promoter, but it also helps your body build up, but more so maintain, a very healthy immune system. If you remember I mentioned antibodies as well as immunoglobulins a few aminos ago, serine helps to produce these disease killers as well!

Speaking really fast about your immune system again, it may seem that serine is an awesome fighter and you may want to start taking it in a supplement form. It'll probably be a good idea to run that by your doctor and maybe have your blood tested for its serine levels first. Having serine levels that are too high may have the opposite effect on your health and really screw your immune system over.

<u>Taurine, Enough Said!</u>

Taurine was actually one of the amino acids I sold regularly as an associate for a nutritional supplement company, and I knew a few things that it did. I also knew it wasn't discussed very often and people would come in just for that from all over our region. It made me actually really study amino acids when I read into it to gain a better understanding of why people wanted it as a supplement as it was a nonessential amino acid. What I read really stole my interest.

You're going to find taurine in high concentrations inside of your heart as well as skeletal muscles. It is also very prevalent in white blood cells as well as being a really hard worker in your central nervous system.

I also found out the importance of taurine by it's relationship to other amino acids. Amino acids are the building blocks of our cells basically, right? Other amino acids depend on taurine to help them develop. Taurine is a building block to other amino acids! I found that extremely interesting and made me wonder if it could be said that taurine is the most essential, nonessential, amino acid in regards to its interaction and relationship with the other aminos.

I digress, let's go back to taurine's importance with the heart muscle (more specifically the heart). Potassium is an important mineral to our heart (among other muscles), and when we are lacking in it we can develop some serious issues, including potentially dangerous heart arrhythmias. Taurine comes into the heart regard for things like atherosclerosis, hypertension, and so on but it also preventing the heart muscle from losing too much potassium.

Potassium isn't the only mineral that finds taurine to be beneficial. In fact, sodium, calcium, and magnesium also need taurine present to be properly utilized.

Leaving minerals, let's go back and discuss the central nervous system briefly. Taurine acts as a protector to your brain especially during times of dehydration. Aside from that, taurine can also be used medically to treat brain issues such as anxiety, epilepsy, brain function in general, hyperactivity, and seizures.

One thing you may know about seizures is that adults have them at a far more common rate than children. This is where a strong correlation comes into play as taurine being considered important for brain health. Children have four times the amount of taurine, as far as concentration, in their brains than adults do. With that being said, there are a lot of questions raised regarding a correlation between taurine deficiencies as well studies being done that are looking into answering taurine's importance in regular/adequate levels in your brain.

What else caused those questions is a mineral known as zinc. Taurine isn't thought to have zinc as a defendant as much as potassium and magnesium for example. However, if you have a taurine as well as a zinc deficiency you may have impaired vision. Taurine deficiencies leading to seizures thus make a taurine deficiency promoting the prevalence of epilepsy a much more real idea.

One last thing I want to get into about taurine before we move on to tyrosine, our last amino acid, is fats. You won't be excited to hear that taurine doesn't metabolize fats or fatty acids as much as other amino acids do, however the conversation of fat does involve taurine! Serum cholesterol levels need to be controlled, taurine helps with that.

Vitamins, specifically fat soluble vitamins, need to be properly absorbed, and taurine helps with that as well, but here's the real fat kicker. Taurine helps your bile by being a key component of it. Bile is what helps your body digest fat, so everything else is able to metabolize it!

The Final Nonessential Amino Acid

Tyrosine is our final nonessential amino acid, if you are reading them in an ABC type of order at least. It's also an extremely important all around amino acid and does quite a few of important tasks.

One important feature of tyrosine that you will find, or at least now will know, is that it helps regulate your metabolism in general (IE it doesn't just help you absorb, digest, metabolize, etc.).

Speaking of metabolism, a side trick that tyrosine can perform is to suppress your appetite! Oh, on top of metabolizing, tyrosine can also help you get rid of body fat!

Tyrosine helps with a few brain, hormone, and mood based elements, want to know how/ It works by attaching itself iodine atoms. What happens when tyrosine attaches to iodine atoms is that you get active thyroid hormones. It's not just the thyroid gland that is helped big time by tyrosine, your body needs tyrosine for your adrenal as well as pituitary glands to work as well.

I mentioned that tyrosine can help in regards to moods, and here's how (this may be beneficial if you suffer depression or anxiety). Tyrosine acts as a precursor to two specific neurotransmitters, norepinephrine as well as dopamine. Those are thought to be key deficiencies in the ongoing investigation into depression and what causes it.

I'll end the conversation on tyrosine by saying it also helps release melanin which dictates the pigments (colors) of your hair and skin color.

Make Sure You Get These: The Essential Amino Acids

The nonessential amino acid section is completed, truthfully there was a lot of good information I'm hoping you picked up on. Although they were nonessential amino acids, you should realize what happens when you don't have enough of them and should have a deeper understanding of what happens when you're not working properly.

Truthfully, that's a small part of why I (this is my choice, I am not encouraging, recommending, or telling you to do this - I am a smart man, not a doctor so no suing) personally rather treat myself and go to the doctors mainly for blood work and to test my oxygen levels.

Your liver needs to be functioning to produce (most) of the nonessential amino acids, you're making them. The essential amino acids MUST be taken in by your diet! These amino acids are NOT produced in your body, and along with phytonutrients, is a core reason you really have to take in as balanced of a diet as possible.

One thing you need to make for certain is that you are not overdoing your essential amino acids through diet. We saw what could happen by over doing a few nonessential amino acids, the adverse effects here are, for a lack of words, just as adverse and detrimental.

Again, I'll be helping you learn about these amino acids in a structured and ABC type order, actually they start with H but I didn't want to add a new technicality to your life.

Everything is so ridiculously technical these days, don't you agree? Let's look at our essential amino acids!

Histidine

Have you ever heard of a myelin sheath? You've read about them briefly in this book so far, but I didn't throw their technical name at you. Myelin sheaths help your body protect the nerve cells from things like free radicals and such. Did you guess I was going to say that histidine is an essential (no pun on words) amino acid in their maintenance? You're wrong! Histidine is important in maintaining your myelin sheaths (notice the word usage?) That was a bad joke, I digress and let's continue.

Along the topic of histidine and cells, your red and white blood cells also find a need for this essential amino acid. Actually, they don't need it so much to function but to come into existence. Your body needs histidine to produce white and red blood cells.

Here's something interesting but I really don't think you want to test. On the same topic of red and white blood cells, there's a belief out there that this amino may actually help prevent AIDS! Again, going out and sharing needles or having unprotected sex is one of the most foolish and reckless things you can do - don't test the theory, science or not.

AIDS kills your immune system and hampers your blood cell counts, this is another area where it is beneficial (and essential) to have histidine in your body. Why am I repeating myself you may be wondering? I'm not, in fact I am about to tell you that histidine helps to create levels of histamine (should have mentioned this is an immune system chemical) in your body.

A cool trick, or ability, that may make your teens want to learn about amino acids is the role this essential player (that's a pun on upcoming words, your teens will get it) has in the sexual arena! Yeah, histidine is an essential amino acid for natural human sexual functions. This "player" has the ability to aid in sexual arousal. Before we go and call this the aphrodisiac of amino acids, I do have to say it also aids in feeling sexual pleasure as well as sexual functioning. Okay, now you can pretty much call it the aphrodisiac of amino acids.

Let's go into the effects of high and low levels in regards to their effects of histidine in your body. High levels of histidine appear to affect your psychological health, while low levels appear to hit you physically.

High levels of histidine are found to be a common trait in people with schizophrenia. One of the side effects of too much histidine is want to take a guess? That's not it, I was trying to give you an opportunity to guess and in turn possibly have your self esteem climb to a slightly higher level because you got an answer correct. So that's your guess? Absolutely, the answer is schizophrenia! How did you guess? Either way, great job.

Schizophrenia from what I've heard from the voices in my head (bad joke, but it made some people laugh, told you I was not politically correct) is not fun at all and can drive you "crazy". I use crazy in an un-literal sense of the word, and stay with me for a second. Anxiety can drive you crazy as well, and that is another trademark condition of your body having too much histidine.

If your body has less than adequate levels of histidine present than you may show signs of something called nerve deafness as well as rheumatic symptoms.

We're into the essential amino acids, and we know we need to take these aminos in through diet or supplements.People with manic depression, also known as bipolar disorder, should not take histidine unless their doctor verifies their levels of this amino are low enough to warrant dietary inclusion.

We know we need histidine as we don't make it in our body, but where can we get it from? There are 3 sources known to give you an adequate supply.

You can find acceptable levels of histidine in rye, wheat, as well as in rice. I have not seen anything convincing that states the type of rice however. My educated guess would be to eat some (good for you) wheat and rye bread.

Isoleucine, Number One!

Are you wondering what I am numbering (aside from isoleucine)? I'm not going onto a rant or anything, alphabetically though, isoleucine is the first of our branched-chain amino acids!

This amino acid is metabolized in your muscle tissue, and goes along with branched-chain amino acids (exactly, because it is one). It aids you therefore in your body maintaining stable levels of energy.

Your body, again, needs you to eat isoleucine for a few good reasons, the first obviously being it releasing energy. The first has to deal with blood, which I've read a few times you need to survive. Hemoglobin is the first thing I mentioned that your body needs in regards to blood and isoleucine helps you to form it. Along with hemoglobin, your body uses this essential amino for blood sugar stabilization. It also helps you to naturally regulate your blood sugar.

With the mentioning of blood sugar stabilization and regulation, you may be wondering if this amino acid is beneficial to those with diabetes. I have been wondering that exact same question for over 4 years now, and have yet to see anything conclusive. I wouldn't take a guess at either yes or no in it being beneficial; I was actually looking into it for individuals labeled as being pre-diabetic. The jury is still out to use a pun, but great mind for wondering. Speaking of minds, let's get into the effects of unbalanced levels of isoleucine and what you really need to take it with for it to work properly.

People with low levels of isoleucine have been found to suffer from a wide range, too wide for the scope of this book (additionally I think there are many contributing additional factors). Effects can be both mental and physical. A deficiency however can be found in people showing signs of hypoglycemia.

So what can we have for dinner that contains isoleucine, let's grab a list:

- Chicken
- Chickpeas
- Eggs
- Fish
- Lentils
- Meat
- Many seeds (there's a bunch of them, many have essential fatty acids as well so eat up!)
- Soy

This is a branched-chain amino, and I will tell you that this is one of the things I personally supplement with so I am taking balanced levels of each BCAA (branched-chain amino acid). Make sure the purity is good on them. You can also visit For the BCAA's I use if you want to take my word for it. Again, please be wise and run this by your doctor first.

Our Second Branched-Chain Amino Acid, Leucine

Leucine is the second alphabetical BCAA, and there's not a tremendous amount of information on it compared with other amino acids. That is by no means a hint toward it being less than important, it is essential for a reason (we need it because we don't make it). But why do we need leucine?

Leucine is instrumental in increasing the production of growth hormone. It also lowers elevated blood sugar. The other portions of it tie in with the complete whole of BCAA's. It also works in conjunction with its BCAA brethren (or sisters depending on if you have feminist beliefs or tendencies, I won't judge).

Working with the other branched-chain aminos leucine helps to act as fuel and protect your muscles. Aside from protecting, they also aid in healing things you've become attached to (literally) like your bones, skin, and muscle tissue.

So what can we chomp on to get this goodness? Again, I'd visit http:sixpackabsv.com/bcaa for some good information on branched-chain amino acid supplements, with that being said you're going to want to supplement to get a balanced effect. However, leucine is also found in varying amounts in the foods listed below:

- BROWN rice (capitalized for a reason)
- Beans

- Various meat
- Nuts
- Soy FLOUR
- Unadulterated whole wheat

Valine, I Broke The Structure

I wanted to keep the branched-chain amino acids in order, and I apologize for that well not really I apologize for breaking up my ABC order. Valine is the third of the BCAAs and again needs to be taken in a balanced conjunction with isoleucine and leucine.

This amino acid can be called a hyperactive essential amino. Your body can use this as an energy source (like [weakly] isoleucine and more so leucine) because of the fact it is a branched-chain amino. Your entire body can't use it as an energy source, but your muscles can.

Being used as an energy source isn't the only reason I call this a hyperactive essential amino acid, if that was the case I would be biased. This amino acid also has a stimulant effect in your body though.

Back to the discussion of muscle, valine helps with other aminos to aid in muscular metabolization. If you're looking for valine you can find high concentrations of it in your muscle tissue, much like glutamine.

Valine isn't just an energy increasing amino acid, it is also very beneficial in helping your body repair damaged tissue.

Valine is also a sort of a resurrection, not in a sense of my Lord Jesus, but in regards to other amino acids. If you abuse drugs, there's a good chance you are going to start depleting amino acids in your body. Drug addiction can cause severe depletion of amino acids. Valine helps to correct this issue.

Don't take too much valien though, it can make you feel like things are crawling on you and there is nothing there! It can also make you "trip" to use a drug addiction reference is basically hallucinations That makes me wonder if too much long term valine can create a nerve issue or even deeply affect your brain chemistry? I haven't seen anything on that but it does make a lot of sense, don't you agree?

You can get valine in supplement form (so you take it in a balanced manner with the other branched-chain amino acids). As far as taking it in through food it can be found in:

- Dairy products
- Grains (a variety have varying, but solid levels)
- Meats
- Mushrooms
- Peanuts
- Soy

Let's get back to our structured method of discussing essential aminos!

Lysine Is A REALLY Cool Amino (See Why)

Lysine is another extremely important amino acid for protein, it is a vital building block in all protein. It's also extremely crucial for your (mainly children's but you need it too) bones. It helps them grown (told you children need it) and properly develop. This could be because it helps with calcium absorption, and speaking of elements allows adults to maintain a good balancing act with nitrogen in their body.

Like every other amino acid, lysine helps in more than one way. Lysine is an amazing producer, and it wears a lot of production hats, meaning it helps to produce a variety of different things. What sort of things does it produce? Antibodies are a good starting point. Lysine also helps with the production of enzymes as well as a variety of hormones. We can also throw in collagen as something it helps to create.

It doesn't just help us form, produce, and absorb it also repairs tissue. Speaking of tissue repair, lysine may be a beneficial supplement for athletes to take. Lysine is able to build muscle protein. Let's expand who this could be good for. What about people recovering from a sports related injury or surgery? They can also be added by taking a lysine supplement!

Let's expand on our expansion here and cover ground we haven't really covered yet. Lysine is also beneficial to people who have issues with herpes (issues meaning they are infected, not because of a misunderstanding. That's an FYI). This is going to include cold sores.

If you want to battle or possibly even prevent a herpes or cold sore outbreak it will be beneficial for you to take your lysine along with vitamin C (make sure it contains bioflavonoids and make sure you read about bioflavonoids in **Phytonutrient Superfoods**). While doing this (fighting the big bad herpes issue) make sure you are avoiding foods rich in arginine!

Aside from L-Lysine supplements, you may be wondering where you can find this essential amino acid because you know you don't make it and you want to ensure you do not become deficient. Here's a list for you:

- Cheese
- Eggs
- Fish
- Lima beans (your childhood arch nemesis)
- Milk
- Potatoes
- RED meat
- Products containing soy
- Yeast

Methionine, Major Essential Amino!

The first time I heard about methionine I read it fast and thought someone was asking me if they should take methadone (a narcotic to help with heroin withdrawals). After rereading their question I told them they definitely want to bring it up to their doctors attention (that they want methionine not that they have a heroin issue). They had good reason for asking about it. They were diagnosed with fatty liver and, well let's look into the benefits of this major amino acid!

In the last paragraph I mentioned a customer that spoke with me regularly online told me they were diagnosed with fatty liver. They saw methionine mentioned numerous times when looking into alternative treatments for the condition and asked me about it. I'll tell you about it too seeing I spent about 3 days researching it for them.

Methionine is extremely important for your liver as well as your body's arteries. One of the most important traits of this essential amino acid is that it helps to prevent a fat build up. A fatty liver could see a reduction in the production of other vital, and bodily created aminos. Too much fat in your blood could end up stopping or greatly reducing the amount of blood flow important organs, such as your kidneys, brain, and your heart. Both of these could cause some serious complications.

Aside from a fat annihilator, methionine also is an extremely potent antioxidant. This essential amino is known to enjoy destroying or neutralizing harmful free radicals.

Another reason methionine is essential is that every single cell in your body absolutely needs it to synthesize and process a variety of things in your body namely nucleic acids, collagen (this amino also helps with nail and skin issues on a more minor level), as well as proteins. Think about that for a second, without methionine your cells can't synthesize proteins which will lead to eventual mutilation of your cells. This is thought to lead to cancer. Cancer leads to an eventual death.

The following part here is going to be broken down and I need you to try and stay with me, this is a potentially difficult to understand, but extremely interesting and important feature of methionine. The more toxins we have in our body, the more we need methionine. Not because methionine attacks the toxins (free radicals however, which are something different it does, attack and neutralize), but toxins attack the liver. Stick with me.

Your liver acts as sort of an incubator or creation center for a variety of amino acids, right? One of the key liver saving amino acids is glutathione, glutathione if memory serves you, you will remember, helps to neutralize and destroy the harmful toxins and protect your liver. If your body is overloaded with toxins, glutathione can become depleted, and this is where methionine comes in.

Let's work backwards and see how methionine is important at indirectly helping your liver in this case. Your body will take methionine and convert it into cysteine. Your body will then take this and use it as a precursor to glutathione and thus build your levels up.

Let's start looking into individuals and conditions that can benefit from supplementally taking methionine (and you should probably have it in your diet, another thing to run by your doctor [if you haven't caught on, before lifestyle or diet changes you need to tell your doctor]). Let's start with how this could help pregnant women (you MUST run this by your doctor!), it could help you prevent or potentially treat rheumatic fever as well as toxemia.

Although "the pill" seems to becoming less popular as other forms of contraceptives are becoming more widespread, women who take the pill may see a benefit from supplemental methionine.

If you're wondering why, and I'd be willing to bet you are (not because I'm an arrogant windbag, this is just something very few people know about) it' because methionine can help their bodies excrete estrogen.

Women aren't the only people who can be benefited greatly by methionine supplementation (remember, we're covering essential amino acids here). Do you remember I mentioned that high levels of histamine can increase the chances of schizophrenia or people with schizophrenia? Methionine can help lower histamine levels in their bodies.

Before we get into another food list, I want to touch on (very briefly, I swear) a brain food source called choline. Choline is derived from methionine, which could thus deplete methionine stores in your body faster.

Let's look at how we can include this particular amino acid in our diet instead of running for the supplement!

- Beans
- Eggs

- Fish
- Garlic (and you can keep Vampires away too!)
- Lentils
- Onions (also a great source of the flavonoids that make up quercetin)
- Soy beans
- A variety of seeds
- Yogurt

The Tongue Twisting Essential Amino Called Phenylalanine

Can you do me a favor and say the name of this essential amino acid 10 times rapid fire? There's something about this amino and i have pronounced it correctly potentially twice in my life. But don't worry, I know all of the important things about it!

Let's start off talking about brains in a familiar fashion. Do you remember where I mentioned your body had a blood-brain barrier that helped protect it from invaders, free radicals, toxins, etc.? You will remember I called a select few amino acids VIPs, phenylalanine is one of those VIPS.

Phenylalanine is important when it comes to your brain because of how it influences part of your brain chemistry. It is also thought that phenylalanine can help with a couple very serious, and one very painful, brain or neurological problems.

Your body uses this tongue twisting amino acid to convert into tyrosine, another amino (nonessential as the body is making it) that has a direct impact on your mood.

We're going to cover a tricky explanation of phenylalanine, the confusing part is that it is created, taken, or used in 3 separate forms. Think of it sort of like a trifecta idea (bad term, but it's not technically a trio either), and each form does something drastically different than the others, except for one of them which appears to be a 1 - 2 punch.

We'll start with the most common form of v, L-phenylalanine. We mentioned proteins need amino acids, right? This is the particular form that is incorporated into your (and mine) body's proteins. The D form isn't directly correlated with your body's proteins, however it does work on the neurological side. The D form is known to act as a painkiller!

The third form of phenylalanine is DL-phenylalanine, and if you took a wild guess and said it is a combination of the L and D forms, you're right! DL-phenylalanine is a really heavy hitter, it helps to control pain (the D form) as well as being a building block to proteins. That isn't all, this form goes a step further and increases your mental alertness, can help to suppress a hungry appetite, and can aid with individuals suffering from Parkinson's disease!

This note is for the guy's. Does your girl suffer from PMS and it drives you crazy? You may tell her from a very safe distance (and if she begins growling or screaming instantly throw chocolate at her) to ask her doctor about DL-phenylalanine as it can aid in alleviating PMS symptoms! Thank me later when your life is slightly less hormonal.

The dietary addition seems to be a lot tougher to gain information on this amino, phenylalanine. I haven't seen adequate amounts of food containing it, thus being said you may want to ask your doctor if a supplement containing it could be beneficial to you.

Threonine

Threonine has some of the least rolls I have come across in my studies into amino acids. I also, when reading about it and studying the why's and how's of aminos, came to the conclusion that this amino is still extremely important. Not because it is an essential amino acid, but because of its huge roles.

Think of threonine as a sort of referee, or quality assurance manager. This essential amino is responsible for maintaining a balance of proteins in your body. Aside form that this is a key precursor to two other amino acids, glycine and taurine.

Aside from being a Q/A manager, threonine also helps your body's immune system. It is thought to help with producing antibodies. On a neurological view (because threonine is found in skeletal muscle, your heart, as well as your central nervous system) it can also aid in alleviating symptoms of some forms of depression.

Threonine is another amino acid I have found to have an inadequate amount of information on, in regards to food. I did however read that vegetarians could be screwed, which led me to believe that meat or fish were a good source of this essential amino acid.

I came to that conclusion by the fact vegetarians do not eat meat or fish (real vegetarians, the other type that eats fish we can call walking animal meat haters, yes?). This may be another amino acid you might want to talk about as being one of your supplements with your doctor.

Tryptophan, My Controversial Amino!

An essential amino acid, is also an illegal amino acid. Do you see why I call it my controversial amino? You may wonder, why talk about something illegal that you can't take? Au contraire!

You can take this amino via diet, you just cannot legally buy a supplement of full blown tryptophan. Let's look into a story of lies, cover up, and murder (LITERALLY, how cool is this amino?)!

Over two decades ago, on a dark dreary day in November of 1989, the Center for Disease Control, a powerful player in American life, reported evidence that L-tryptophan caused eosinophilia myalgia syndrome (it is just as bad as it sounds) they started encouraging people to run from the supplement. After that, all supplement form L-tryptophan were ordered shot dead instantly.

Although they may not have been shot dead, some supplements did actually cause death. L-tryptophan? No, not the supplement per say but actually contaminants inside the product caused the deadly syndrome. So go and buy some l-tryptophan. Wait, you can't as it is still banned in the USA.

BUT WE CAN GET IT FROM FOOD SO LET'S GO ON! How was that story? As you can tell, fiction isn't my strongest point so we'll get back into fact, sound good? Your brain uses tryptophan to help it create serotonin (not an amino acid, but it is an important neurotransmitter!).

Your body uses the tryptophan influenced creation to transfer impulses between nerves (think of it as an internal conversation on the nerve level).

Actually, I almost named this my "sleepy amino" because this particular amino acid that creates serotonin can be called being responsible for sleep. If you suffer from depression, insomnia or even mild sleeplessness tryptophan may be beneficial. This amino is even known to aid in helping to stabilize moods!

Some people that could be helped by tryptophan are hyperactive children. Where this amino (well, the serotonin it creates) can help with depression, it also helps decrease hyperactivity.

Insufficient levels of tryptophan could actually really screw up your levels of serotonin, and if you're on the low side of both magnesium as well as tryptophan you could be looking at coronary artery spasms (trust me, I doubt they're fun).

Seeing you can't get the supplement for tryptophan, where will you be able to get more into your diet? Start by eating a diet that consists (obviously among other things) of:

- BROWN rice (capped for a reason)
- Cottage cheese
- Meat
- Peanuts
- And Protein (mainly soy protein)

The End.....? NOPE!

We're done, right? We've covered inside and out pretty much everything you need to know about amino acids, right? Well you are correct, but are we done? No way! You have a bonus section of "close but not an amino" nutrients, and you're going to love the power inside of these guys! I'd highly encourage you to talk to your doctor about maybe supplementing with these along with the essential amino acids! Here we go!

A Non-Amino Powerhouse and A Fat Person's New Best Friend, Carnitine

Carnitine has long been one of my favorite amino acids to read about for a variety of reasons. Alright, maybe just because it's really interesting! Carnitine has a similar structure to amino acids and is normally considered to actually be an amino but it isn't. You can call it a cousin of the aminos (which interesting carnitine is actually a B vitamin substance!)

If you remember real, or true, amino acids have the ability and need to synthesize proteins and/or act as neurotransmitters. Not carnitine, this is where carnitine had helped me become a notoriously awesome sales associate for the vitamin chain I mentioned I worked at for a while. Carnitine is fat's worst enemy on a few levels.

First, the most popular fat fighting function of carnitine is that it doesn't let fat get stored in your body. It beats your fat and then transport the long-chain fatty acids to be used as an energy source by the mitochondria in your body.

The effect of this is the second and less direct level of carnitine's fight against fat. If the fat isn't being stored and is being used to provide energy, your heart, liver (that produces the nonessential aminos aside from those that are created by other aminos), and muscle!

Another thing that carnitine can help with, and this one hits home with me personally is the third way it deals with fat, and that is to help alleviate symptoms of chronic fatigue syndrome. I will tell you CFS sucks, bad. It can literally suck your life away. How do I know? I had signs of it for years.

I just mentioned, and thus you should have just learned (if not reread it, really cool stuff) a few paragraphs ago that carnitine helps by pretty much spoon feeding your mitochondria. There's a large belief that a lot of the CFS issues stem from a disruption in your mitochondria and how they release or absorb energy (I've seen it go both ways quite often, to me it's inconclusive). This is thought to be a huge factor in the fatigue.

One thing I read when I was suffering bad (I should disclose my diet sucked for a large lack of words) is that people with CFS had greatly decreased levels of carnitine. I used myself as a guinea pig and, well legally I can't nor would I (as my doctor was unsure) say I am cured but I will say I feel amazing now. Could it have been diet? Maybe. Could it have been the L-carnitine supplement I was popping a few times a day feeding fatty acids (long-chained) to my mitochondria? Maybe.

Another major problem in our country is diabetes. I'm not going to say carnitine can help directly with diabetes, but I have read in quite a few sources that a trademark issue caused by diabetes is improper fat metabolism. Carnitine could help wit the health risks associated with this issue.

Carnitine is not just a fat (and I'll throw in triglyceride) enemy, it's a friend to antioxidant super powers! Specifically vitamins C and E. What carnitine does with these two vitamins is to help your natural aging process come to a screeching halt. Maybe not that extreme, but it does slow it down tremendously.

Another cool thing about carnitine as compared to true amino acids (although I would argue about this to potentially include glutamine) is the fact they differ in the fact aminos are more equal whereas carnitine has a bias. We mentioned we all make some levels of carnitine, but it seems carnitine can occur more (or in higher levels) in women than in men! This is because of the muscle mass, making a nonhereditary deficiency of carnitine more likely in men.

If you think men have it bad, you should feel bad for vegetarians as opposed to their non vegetarian counterparts. The reason for this one is that plant protein does not contain carnitine. Additionally, methionine and lysine are not found in plant protein either which means carnitine has a better chance at not being found in a vegetarian (which if vampires went after carnitine levels instead of blood, vegetarians would naturally feel safe).

To offset this issue, a vegetarian or vegan could eat something like cornmeal or other grains that have been fortified with lysine. I can gladly say, I do not have a carnitine issue because I would never eat that vegan meat substitute (nasty, nasty tasting stuff. I did in fact vomit) and if a vegetarian or vegan doesn't like cornmeal a carnitine supplement will always be another option.

Your body can make carnitine if you have proper amounts of iron, thiamine (B1), pyridoxine (B6), lysine, and methionine. Just because you can make it doesn't mean your body can synthesize it. For that to happen you also need adequate vitamin C levels.

Something you may find interesting is that a carnitine deficiency can actually be due to your genes!

Carnitine is normally found inside of meat.

Just like phenylalanine, carnitine comes in a few different forms supplementally. You'll find D, L, and DL (this one can make you sick, I'd stay away unless told otherwise) forms of carnitine available as well as Acetyl-L-Carnitine.

ALC (acetyl-l-carnitine) is actually just as cool as carnitine is, I'll cover a few reasons why. Like carnitine, ALC (a carnitine derivative) is produced in the body (vegetarians are screwed here again) and acts mildly similar.

If you're dieting or trying to eat healthier ALC may become your little dieting buddy! Like carnitine this non-amino but awesome runner up can deal with fats and bring them into the mitochondria for energy, but it also plays with the synthesis of protein as well as carbohydrates! Let's look at this and why it's important for you.

As I mentioned your body can benefit from carnitine (and now you know ALC as well) bringing fat to your mitochondria, but why's that so important? There are 3 main sources your muscle and body can use as energy, fats, carbohydrates, and protein.

There's a tossup of whether it is more important for your body to use fat or carbohydrates as a primary energy source, but regardless you want protein to be used to do all of the other immensely important jobs it has. So when you have carnitine and it's derivative ALC bringing fats to your mitochondria, you're standing a better chance at allowing protein to do what it needs to do.

Getting back to ALC, did you know it is one of the more studied compounds that we know about? The reason for that is that ALC has some superior antiaging properties.

Science has found and accepted that sometimes ALC has the ability to prevent, slow down and (potentially, I am not convinced completely, neither is science) begin reversing neurological (brain) and nervous system degeneration.

There have been numerous studies into daily supplementation and its amazing slow down of the effects and progression of Alzheimer's disease. It has been shown in studies to lessen the deterioration of memory, attention, spatial abilities, as well as language. Is it a cure? No, but in regards to things like Alzheimer's any family member will tell you a little bit of help at all is a gift from God.

I have been reading into some studies that are showing a correlation between the benefits of ALC and its effect on dementia, and mood based disorders such as some forms of depression. Again, and your doctor will say this, the benefits help treatment but no study has shown them to be cures.

We're not done with what benefits ALC has on your body, it's helping power for a lack of words, can also be seen in how it can enhance the immune system as well as slow cerebral aging (anti aging) and stimulate certain enzymes to act as antioxidants.

I mentioned how carnitine can aid in some ailments caused by a diabetic condition, ALC is thought to as well! It is thought that ALC can potentially prevent nerve damage commonly associated with diabetes!

Do you remember when I said that branched-chain amino acids can be beneficial to those who exert stress (athletes, I wanted to be fancy)? ALC can enhance the performance benefits of BCAAs as well!

I told you that these were some cool almost aminos didn't I! I don't lie, the information above I have seen firsthand was life changing to some individuals.

With that information being said, I had seen many times this had helped individuals while working in the nutritional supplement store, I have also seen times stopping a medical treatment and jumping right in to ALC supplementation instead had adverse effects.

It is imperative that you speak with your doctor. Remember I do not go regularly to a doctor, however I cannot do my own blood tests or test my own oxygen. I personally feel it is an unwise move, especially if you have any condition, to stop seeing a doctor.

I'm a huge fan of amino acids, and in fact at social gatherings I have no problem talking about them. Being said, I really am fun to be around and my children absolutely love me! I like to talk about amino acids, because I truly have a love for helping people and that has turned into an obsession of sorts.